THE COMPLETE STRETCHING EXERCISE FOR

MEN OVER 50

Unleash Your Vitality, Mobility, Stay Active, and Embrace Life, Stretching Exercise Tailored for vibrant Seniors.

Cynthia j spencer DPT

Copyright©2023 Cynthia j spencer DPT

Dedication

I dedicate this book to my understanding husband, who took out his time to give me every support I needed for the success of this book, and also to my beautiful kids, who *also played a big role in being patient with me during the time this masterpiece of "**the complete stretching exercise for men over 50**" was being created. I love you all.you mean the world to me*

Table Of Contents

Chapter 1: Getting Started.

How to Use This Book

Congratulations for deciding to use "The Complete Stretching Exercise for Men Over 50" to improve your health and well-being! You'll find a variety of stretches in this book that are especially meant for men who are over fifty. To help you get the most out of this priceless resource, follow these steps:

1. Familiarise Yourself with the Book:

Spend some time reading the introduction to learn about the goals and advantages of stretching exercises for men who are over 50. Recognize how crucial it is to keep your mobility and flexibility as you age.

2. Assess Your Current Fitness Level:

Prior to beginning the exercises, assess your flexibility and range of motion. This will enable you to monitor your development over time and decide where to start. Examine any particular places that could need more care since they are stiff or have less movement.

3. Follow the Instructions:

For every stretching exercise, carefully follow the directions provided. Make sure you are aware of the proper breathing exercises, posture, and length of time for each stretch. Maintaining good form is essential to maximizing the advantages and preventing injuries.

4. Start with the Basics:

It is best to start with the fundamental stretches described in the book if you are new to stretching or haven't worked out in a long time. These stretches will help prevent muscular strains by introducing your body to stretching on a gentle level. As you gain comfort, gradually increase the level of difficulty.

5. Create a Stretching Routine:

Create a stretching regimen that works for your objectives and schedule. Choose if you'd rather stretch in the morning to get your day going or in the evening to wind down and relax. Aim for at least three stretching sessions per week because consistency is essential.

6. Warm Up Before Stretching:

It is crucial to allow your muscles to warm up before beginning any stretching activities. Before stretching, spend five to ten minutes doing a modest aerobic activity, such as brisk walking or cycling, to improve blood flow and prime your body for maximum flexibility.

7. Listen to Your Body:

During the stretches, be aware of any pain or discomfort you may experience. Although stretching should be difficult at times, it should never hurt. To prevent damage, modify the stretches' duration or intensity as necessary. If you have any questions or concerns about pre-existing conditions, speak with a healthcare provider.

8. Track Your Progress:

To track your progress, use the tracking pages included in the book or keep a notebook. Take note of any gains in mobility, flexibility, and general wellbeing. This will act as a powerful incentive to keep you dedicated to your stretching regimen.

Keep in mind that the book "The Complete Stretching Exercise for Men Over 50" is an important tool that can improve your general health and energy. Go slowly, stay steady, and enjoy the process as you work toward more adaptability and a higher standard of living. Cheers to your happy extending!

INTRODUCTION

"Life is movement." During my first semester of graduate school, I heard an old-school chiropractor say these words. These words now have more significance for me as an amateur athlete and doctor who practises physical medicine. Providing daily pain relief to patients has reaffirmed for me the value of mobility in both my personal and professional life.

After 25 years of experience, I've learned that effective and targeted stretching is the key to leading an active, pain-free, and productive life. Regular stretching can lead to a happier, more balanced life.

I've been listening to my patients for a while now as they talk about their experiences with chronic pain while they go about their daily lives. They talk about how difficult it is for them to get out of bed in the morning, how uncomfortable it is for them to get in and out of their cars, how their prolonged desk work strains their shoulders and backs, and how their constant texting causes stiff hands and necks.

The sedentary lifestyle of today is a contributing factor to many of these chronic illnesses. I've discovered that stretching is the most affordable, practical, and safe type of exercise that anyone can do to enhance their general physical health. Emotional well-being is correlated with improved physical and general health.

For individuals with varying degrees of physical fitness, Stretching for Beginners is an excellent tool. Each exercise's thorough instructions and pictures walk you through safely and effectively stretching the targeted muscles.

This simple guide can help you reach your goals by improving your flexibility and reducing discomfort and soreness, whether you are new to stretching, starting a new fitness regimen, or recuperating from an injury or illness.

With this book, I hope to give you a foundation for using good stretching to enhance your physical and mental well-being. You will discover the advantages of stretching, the science underlying it, and safe stretching techniques in part 1.

Learn how to stretch and how to breathe correctly as part of your everyday routine. Go to part 1, chapter 3 if you want to get started straight away.

I tried to keep things easy in this book because there are so many various kinds of stretching techniques that are popular in the media.

Therefore, I have restricted the range of stretches to four fundamental types: static or dynamic, which refers to movement with or without movement, and passive or active, which refers to movement with or without external force. When most people think of stretching, they most often think of static stretching, which includes things like touching your toes and maintaining the position.

Part 2 of this book contains key stretches arranged according to several anatomical locations, indicating the targeted muscles for each stretch. Every chapter concentrates on a different part of your body, ranging from your feet to your neck and core. The advantages of each exercise are briefly summarised, along with the kinds of activities or conditions that the stretch is most beneficial for.

To ensure that you complete the stretches correctly, each one also comes with detailed instructions that are illustrated with an easy-to-follow picture. After you're comfortable with the stretches, you can attempt the exercises in section 3. There are programs for general stretches, targeted injuries, and particular sports.

Think carefully before you begin: Before starting any new fitness program, consult your doctor and give yourself a check-up. Be sincere with yourself and reasonable in your aspirations. You'll see results if you make steady, decent progress. Stretch long, stretch slowly, and stretch steadily as a general rule of thumb. Prepare to embark on a journey towards a healthier version of yourself.

WHY STRETCH?

Stand up and give yourself some stretches! Stretching is a great exercise that you can do virtually anywhere and at any time. Spending too much time at your desk? Stand up and give yourself some stretches.

Do you feel stiff and lethargic?
Stand up and give yourself some stretches.
One of the easiest and most beneficial workouts you can do is stretching. Stretching on a regular basis can improve circulation, muscle function, and flexibility; it can also ease mental tension and boost general well-being.

Whether you're an avid fitness enthusiast, a couch potato, or somewhere in between, you'll discover that when you start stretching on a daily basis, your movements will become more fluid and effortless.

Stretching for Beginners might assist all of you beginners who want to have a more flexible physique in reaching your objective. You can change your life, one stretch at a time and one step at a time: A flexible physique and a balanced existence are what you can look forward to when you wave goodbye to tense muscles and creaky joints.

THE MUSCLES

The three main muscle types in the human body are skeletal, smooth, and cardiac. Smooth muscle surrounds the other internal organs, while cardiac muscle is specific to the heart; both forms of muscle are controlled involuntarily and are outside the purview of this book.

Conversely, skeletal muscles are the most prevalent in the body and can be deliberately regulated. Because they aid in holding your skeleton's bones together, these muscles are known as skeletal muscles. Stretching before a workout routine activates your skeletal muscles.

What precisely occurs in your muscles during a stretch? Consider a muscle as an umbrella that can fold up or a telescoping pole: A number of interlocking segments can be extended to lengthen the pole; the segments can be collapsed into themselves to shorten the pole. Muscles behave similarly as they lengthen and contract. Muscle fibre bundles, or big cells, make up a single muscle.

These fibres are composed of stacked units called sarcomeres, which are cylindrical bundles of protein filaments called myosin and actin. Myosin and actin filaments are triggered by calcium ions to glide past one another, shortening the sarcomeres' length in a manner akin to a telescoping pole, which causes muscle contraction. The actin and myosin filaments glide apart during muscular relaxation and elongation, resulting in the lengthening of the sarcomere units.

It's critical to keep in mind that muscles don't move independently. Instead, moving a muscle also moves the corresponding bone and joint.

Tendons, the strong tissue that connects muscle to bone, are where muscles often attach. Ligaments create a capsule-shaped junction by wrapping around the joint and joining two bones.

A sticky substance found in joint capsules lubricates the bones. A muscle that is stretched pulls on a bone and causes the corresponding joint to move.
Your range of motion in your joints is therefore improved by stretching the relevant muscles. Additionally, you improve the blood flow to the joint capsules, which keeps the muscles and joint healthier by supplying more oxygen and nutrients to the area.

Your body's muscles move in relation to where they are located. A muscle has two points of attachment to a bone: its genesis and its insertion. The moveable portion of a muscle contraction is the insertion, and the muscle origin acts as an anchor at a permanent attachment place. A muscle pulls in the direction of its origin from the point of insertion. A muscle's origin is often found closest to the body in relation to its insertion.

Muscle motions are frequently characterized as opposing pairs. Flexion and extension are the most fundamental of them. When a joint flexes, the angle between the bones is reduced; when a joint extends, the angle between the bones is increased. For instance, you are flexing your muscles when you bend your elbow to execute a bicep curl. You are stretching the joint when you flex your elbow and bring your forearm down.

Adduction and abduction make up another directional duo. A limb is moved away from the body's vertical centerline during abduction, much like when you raise your leg out to the side.

A bodily portion that moves toward the vertical centerline is called an adduction. A bone can rotate either internally or externally along its long axis. The movement is internal if the rotation is made in the direction of the body's vertical midline. On the other hand, an external rotation takes place when the movement happens away from the body's vertical midline.

finally, twisting a body component out or in, like when moving your foot, is described by the antagonistic pairs of pronation and supination.

Stretching for Beginners provides a variety of stretching exercises that combine all the fundamental muscle motions and target the key muscle groups of the arms, legs, shoulders, core, and neck.

THE STUDIES

Your body was meant to be mobile. Physiotherapists who research the benefits of movement, such as stretching, consistently come to the same conclusion: by improving cardiovascular function, promoting flexibility, and hastening the healing process after injuries, regular muscle stretching can significantly enhance your quality of life. These are just a few instances of recent stretching-related scientific studies.

Increased Flexibility in the Hamstrings

According to a 2016 study published in the Journal of Physical Therapy Science, participants' hip proprioception and hamstring flexibility increased after seven days of self-myofascial release stretching for 15 minutes each. 1.

Improved Heart Health

Stretching is a useful treatment for enhancing heart rate and cardiovascular health, according to a 2019 study published in the Journal of Strength and Conditioning Research. According to preliminary studies, stretching improves nitric oxide bioavailability, baroreflex sensitivity, and relaxation—all of which may be beneficial for heart health. 2 Improved Equilibrium in the Elderly

Demographic

According to a 10-week study that was published in the International Journal of Health Sciences in 2016, a lower-limb stretching regimen can help older adults maintain better balance, which reduces their risk of falls and injuries. Thirty patients underwent a regimen consisting of static stretching for thirty seconds on the hamstrings, gastrocnemius, and hip flexors. 3 Boosts Muscle Performance According to a 2016 study published in MOJ Yoga and Physical Therapy, young adult athletes' hamstring and quadriceps' strength was enhanced when they preceded more strenuous activity with dynamic stretching movements like butt kicks and straight leg kicks. 4 Better Recovery for Hamstring Strains

Sports injuries and other physical activity frequently result in hamstring strains.

An eight-week study on dancers with hamstring injuries using active and static stretches as well as other range-of-motion therapies was carried out in 2017. The findings, which were published in The Journal of Sports Medicine and Physical Fitness, suggest that stretching therapy can aid with pain management, muscle function enhancement, and increased flexibility.

Enhanced Adaptability in Golfers

A 2018 study that was published in the Journal of Exercise Physiology Online looked at 95 golfers' flexibility throughout the course of a golf season. The findings show that golfers' flexibility in their ankles, lumbar spines, and shoulders is enhanced by stretch exercise. Six

Anyone's quality of life can be improved by regular stretching, regardless of age, activity level, or sedentary lifestyle. Although most individuals are aware that stretching increases range of motion and flexibility, stretching has many other benefits as well. Stretching increases circulation, lessens lower back discomfort and muscular soreness, reduces the risk of injury, expedites the healing process, eases tension and promotes sleep, corrects posture and coordination, boosts performance in sports and sexual activities, and slows the ageing-related loss of physical fitness.

Stretching is a fantastic complimentary activity to strength training and cardiovascular conditioning, and it provides a lot of benefits.

Rises Range of Motion and Flexibility

Stretching improves flexibility, allowing your joints to move through their full range of motion. Stiff joints and taut muscles can make it uncomfortable to do daily tasks. For example, tight hip flexors or shortened calf muscles might make it difficult to climb stairs. You can improve your general mobility by lengthening tense muscles and activating the corresponding joints.

Lessens Pain and Damage

Stretching regularly can help keep your joints and muscles flexible and lower your chance of injury. Tiny microtears in your muscles might end up causing more damage and lead to discomfort and injury if you don't maintain your body flexible.

Fibrotic adhesions, which prevent muscles from correctly elongating, can form on muscle fibers. (picture a kink along the telescoping mechanism of muscle filaments). Being flexible greatly reduces your risk of pulling a muscle during a quick action. This is particularly valid for athletes like tennis or soccer players.

Speeds Recovery

After an injury or surgery, the affected area may be immobilized for a time.
The lack of use and the build-up of collagen leads to a tightening of the
muscles. Stretching helps soften the cross-fiber formation of scar tissue so
The muscle tissue can be restored to normal function.

Boosts Circulation

Muscles behave like vascular pumps when they contract and relax. It's like trying to squeeze a sponge: Squeezing a damp sponge causes fluid to escape; when the sponge relaxes, the fluid returns.

In a similar vein, when you fully extend your muscles, blood passes through the muscle's belly and lubricates the joint as a whole. Blood flow provides oxygen and nutrients to the muscle tissue, which are essential for the muscle's health and function. The metabolic waste produced by using muscles is then removed by the fluid. A muscle that is stretched correctly has the right quantity of blood flowing through it, which lessens the strain on the associated joint and may stop excessive wear and tear.

<u>Ways to Combat a Sedentary Lifestyle</u>

Long hours are frequently required of you in the modern lifestyle, whether you are standing or sitting at a desk. The healthy operation of muscles and joints is negatively impacted by immobility. This lifestyle choice has been linked to a number of neck, shoulder, and back issues. In a similar vein, playing video games or watching TV are examples of contemporary entertainment that exacerbates chronic weariness. Long stretches or periods of sitting still might have negative effects that can be mitigated with specific stretching exercises.

Prior to or following a workout?

Although there are obvious general benefits to stretching, does it really matter how you stretch? The advantages of stretching before or after intense exercise are a topic of much discussion.

You should warm up your muscles with dynamic stretches that resemble the main movements of your workout before beginning a vigorous exercise program. The goal is to increase blood flow to your muscles so they are ready for action. You run the risk of aggravating even the smallest muscle strain if you forget to stretch. Consider the blood in your body as the oil in your car's engine: just as an engine needs to warm up before it can operate correctly, so too do your muscles and joints need to be lubricated before a workout. Enhanced blood circulation to your muscles facilitates more effective, secure, and optimal movement.

Static stretches increase the muscles' stretchability and, eventually, range of motion after a strenuous workout while they are warm and flexible.

<u>Enhances Posture and Diminishes Back Pain</u>

From a biomechanical perspective, excessive muscular contraction during rest might alter postural alignment and result in back pain.

For example, you may lengthen the pectoral muscles in your chest to correct slouched shoulders. Abnormally tightened hamstrings and restricted hip range of motion are frequently linked to chronic back pain. Stretching these areas appropriately may help reduce back discomfort.

Enhances Sleep and Calms the Body

Stretching helps reduce stress because it has a calming effect on both the body and the mind. Stretching exercises probably have a calming effect because they activate the muscles' stretch receptors. You're more likely to get a good night's sleep when you're more at ease.

HOW TO STRETCH

One of the simplest exercises to learn is stretching. Anybody can benefit from a new stretching program, regardless of age or fitness level. Once you adhere to these basic safety and technique standards, you'll be prepared to begin your new workout regimen.

WHAT MAKES A GOOD STRETCH?

Make an Evaluation of Yourself

When you start a new stretching regimen, you probably have a certain objective in mind. The last thing you want to do is injure yourself and make your attempts to enhance your flexibility, posture, or general health ineffective. Therefore, the first thing to do before starting a stretching routine is to evaluate your physical state. Obtain a doctor's clearance if you have any major underlying medical conditions, such as arthritis or heart disease. Additionally, be sincere with yourself and assess yourself: In terms of motion patterns, which parts of your body are the most dysfunctional? What areas of weakness do you have the most?

Target individual muscles within the bigger afflicted muscle groups after addressing the major damaged muscle groups.

Do a Reality Check

You're probably not stretching if it doesn't hurt a little bit.

Recognize your boundaries and learn to pay attention to the messages that your body is sending you.

<u>Establish sensible objectives</u>

Be patient; you are most likely not a professional athlete. Over time, set yourself some reasonable objectives. Let's take an example where you can currently only reach your knees and would like to be able to touch your toes comfortably. In a few weeks, aim to reach the middle of your shins, and celebrate your little victories. Consider this a marathon rather than a sprint. Proceed steadily and slowly.

Get warmed up

When you're ready to start your first stretching routine, make sure your muscles are warmed up. For example, avoid stretching as soon as you wake up if your muscles are still chilly. It's not a good idea to stretch if your muscles aren't sufficiently lubricated. Simple movements cause microtears in everyone's muscles, and if you exercise when your muscles are cold, a tiny microtear could develop into more significant injury. Stretching in the morning can be beneficial if you take a hot shower to increase blood flow.

Hold for Appropriate Length of Time

You must maintain the position for at least 15 to 30 seconds in order for a stretch to be beneficial.

According to several studies, holding the stretch for 30 to 60 seconds has a greater advantage for the elderly population. For as long as it doesn't make you dizzy, you can hold the stretch for a minute.

Inhale!

This may seem apparent, but you risk forgetting to breathe if you're focusing too much on getting into a particular position. Your brain will receive less oxygen if you hold your breath while stretching.
It can make you dizzy or faint. Throughout the stretch, make an effort to breathe constantly by taking slow, deep breaths in and out.

Choose the Appropriate Frequency

For a few weeks, start stretching three or four times a week. Increase the frequency gradually as you advance and as your body adjusts. Pay attention to your body; it will communicate with you. Stop if something hurts. You should be able to distinguish between genuine pain and just minor discomfort.

Maintain Consistency

Find a few minutes each day to allocate the proper amount of work and requirements to each stretch. Remember that doing fewer stretches correctly is preferable to doing too many in a hurry.

Strive for Proper Form

To achieve a proper stretch, generally focus on the muscles for a long, slow, progressive stretch. Any jerky, abrupt movement might cause discomfort or harm. It is unproductive for many beginners to bounce through a stretch. You deny your muscles an opportunity to function at the molecular, neurological, or chemical levels when you bounce. You must give the brain enough time to respond in a way that causes the muscle to relax.

Chapter 1: Getting Started.

The Importance of Warming Up Properly

Regardless of age, stretching is a crucial part of a good warm-up regimen. It becomes even more important for men over 50, though, as it enhances joint health overall and increases flexibility and mobility. The body can experience major changes as we age, such as decreased muscular suppleness, increased stiffness, and an increased chance of injury. Men over 50 must therefore prioritize stretching in order to counteract these consequences and preserve their physical health.

Increased flexibility is one of the main advantages of stretching for men over 50. The ability of muscles and joints to move through their whole range of motion is referred to as flexibility. Age-related muscular atrophy causes constriction and decreased range of motion. Stretching on a regular basis improves range of motion, increases blood flow, and lessens the effects of muscle stress. Improved flexibility not only helps with daily tasks but also improves exercise performance and lowers the possibility of sprains or rips.

Additionally, stretching promotes joint health, which is crucial as men age. Osteoarthritis and other disorders can result from the degeneration of the cartilage that cushions the joints over time. Men over 50 can decrease joint stiffness, enhance synovial fluid production, and improve joint lubrication by performing stretching activities on a regular basis. By doing these steps, you can lessen the strain on your joints and lower your chance of developing age-related joint issues.

Stretching has advantages for the body, but it also improves mental health. Men may grow more stressed, anxious, or depressed as they age for a variety of reasons, including retirement, losing loved ones, or health issues. Doing stretches provides a chance to practice awareness and calm. Stretching facilitates relaxation, stress reduction, and an enhanced sense of wellbeing by releasing tension from the body and mind.

It's crucial to concentrate on a range of muscle groups when doing stretching exercises for guys over 50. Stretches for the neck, shoulders, arms, chest, back, hips, legs, and ankles can be part of this. Given that older muscles may be more prone to damage, it is imperative to pay attention to your body and refrain from overstretching. Increasing flexibility can be accomplished by using static stretches, which include holding a stretch posture for a certain amount of time. The body can benefit from dynamic stretching, which involves extending muscles and joints through their complete range of motion, to warm up and get ready for physical activity.

Before beginning any stretching practice, it is advised to speak with a skilled fitness trainer or healthcare provider, particularly if you have any pre-existing medical ailments or concerns. They may offer you tailored counsel and assist you in creating a stretching regimen that meets your individual requirements.

In summary, males over 50 should stretch frequently to maintain joint health, increase flexibility, and improve general wellbeing. Men can enhance their overall physical performance and lower their chance of injury by adding stretching activities to their warm-up regimen. To make sure you're stretching safely and properly, keep in mind to pay attention to your body, be consistent, and seek professional advice.

Stretching Guidelines and Safety Precautions.

Any fitness program must include stretching since it increases flexibility, reduces risk of injury, and boosts output. However, when performing stretching exercises, it's crucial to adhere to the recommended instructions and take all required safety precautions. The following are some essential rules to remember:

1. Get warmed up Before Stretching: It's important to warm up your muscles and improve blood flow before you stretch. For five to ten minutes, perform mild aerobic exercises like jumping jacks or running. Stretching lessens the chance of strains and pulls by warming up the muscles.

2. Pay Attention to Dynamic Stretching:

Dynamic stretching entails extending the range of motion of the muscles and joints. It aids in warming up the body and energising the muscles in preparation for more strenuous action. Arm circles, leg swings, and walking lunges are a few types of dynamic stretches.

3. Refrain from Stretching Cold Muscles:

It's crucial to refrain from stretching without first warming up since cold muscles are more prone to injury. A warm-up should be performed on your body before beginning any stretching exercises.

4. extend Both Sides:

To keep your balance and prevent muscular imbalances, it's critical to extend your body evenly on both sides. For instance, be sure to stretch your left hamstring in addition to your right.

5. Gradual Progression: It's important to gradually increase the length and intensity of stretches when performing them. Stretching too hard might result in injuries such as tears in the muscles. Stretch lightly at first, then progressively increase the difficulty as you go.

6. Hold Each Stretch: When doing static stretches, hold each one without bouncing for 15–30 seconds. Bouncing has the potential to tighten muscles and raise the danger of harm. Recall to relax into the stretch and take long breaths.

7. Stretch All important Muscle Groups: Pay close attention to stretching the muscles in your neck, shoulders, chest, back, arms, hips, thighs, calves, and ankles, among other important muscle groups. This will lessen the possibility of imbalances and increase general flexibility.

It's crucial to take the following safety measures in addition to adhering to these stretching rules in order to prevent injuries:

1. Listen to Your Body: When you stretch, pay attention to the cues your body gives you. If you feel severe pain or discomfort, stop the stretch right away. Injuries might result from attempting to endure pain.

2. Refrain from Overstretching: Excessive stretching can be detrimental even while it is good. Steer clear of pushing your body above its natural range of motion or excessive stretching. The muscles and connective tissues may be strained as a result.

3. Don't Stretch Injured Muscles: It's advisable to wait to stretch until you've fully healed if you have a strained muscle or another injury. Stretching injured muscles can make them worse and take longer to heal.

4. Speak with a Professional: It is best to speak with a licensed fitness expert or healthcare provider if you have any specific questions or concerns about proper stretching practices. They can offer tailored counsel and direction according to your particular requirements.

You may boost your overall workout performance, lower your chance of injury, and efficiently increase your flexibility by adhering to these stretching rules and safety considerations. Always put safety first and pay attention to your body's limitations. Cheers to your happy extension!

Recommended Equipment for Effective Stretching for Men Over 50.

Stretching is crucial to preserving your aging body's flexibility, mobility, and general health. It's crucial for men over 50 to select the appropriate equipment to improve the efficiency and security of their stretching exercises. Here are a few suggested pieces of equipment:

1. Yoga Mat: For your stretching activities, a good non-slip yoga mat offers a stable and comfortable surface. When doing floor-based stretches, it helps to cushion your joints and keep you from slipping.

2. Foam Roller: Foam rollers are great instruments for self-myofascial release (SMR), which increases flexibility and eases tense muscles. To target particular muscle areas and encourage relaxation, use a foam roller.

3. Stretching Strap: Also known as a yoga strap, a stretching strap is an adaptable tool that helps you reach farther into your stretches, increasing your flexibility. It helps release tense muscles, particularly in the shoulders and lower body.

4. Resistance Bands: These may be used for both strengthening and stretching workouts, and they are available in a variety of strengths. They give your motions resistance, which enhances range of motion and increases muscle endurance.

5. <u>Stability Ball</u>: Using a stability ball might make your stretching exercises more difficult. It improves flexibility and core stability for balance. Stretching with a stability ball works several different muscle groups at once.

6. <u>Balance Board</u>: Using a balance board enhances your body's awareness of its place in space and stability. Stretching using a balancing board improves flexibility and strengthens your lower body and core.

7. <u>Pilates Ring</u>: Also referred to as a magic circle, a Pilates ring can offer support and resistance when performing stretching exercises. It is beneficial to target certain muscle groups, especially the core and upper body.

8. <u>Massage Balls</u>: Used for self-massage and trigger point therapy, massage balls are small, firm balls. By rolling them over your muscles, you may reduce stress and improve blood flow, both of which support the flexibility and health of your tissues.

Keep in mind that when using stretching equipment, safety and appropriate technique are essential. Begin with lower resistance levels and work your way up as your strength and flexibility increase. Before starting any new stretching routine, always get advice from a medical practitioner or trained trainer, especially if you have any prior injuries or medical concerns.

The Role of Flexibility in Fitness for Men Over 50.

All ages should prioritise fitness, but as men become older—50 and beyond—preserving and increasing their flexibility becomes crucial to a well-rounded exercise program. Your muscles and joints' range of motion is referred to as your flexibility. In daily tasks like bending, reaching, and maintaining good posture, it is essential. Men typically get less flexible as they age because of things like diminished suppleness, immobility in the joints, and stiffer muscles. However, you can minimise these impacts and improve your general health and well-being by including flexibility exercises in your workout routine.

Preventing injuries is one of the key advantages of flexibility training for men over 50. Age-related stiffening of the muscles and joints increases the likelihood of sprains, strains, and other injuries. Your body's capacity to move more freely and the possibility of harm from simple acts like bending over to pick something up can both be improved with more flexibility. Due to its ability to increase joint mobility and decrease stiffness, flexibility exercises can also help relieve joint discomfort brought on by diseases like arthritis.

Keeping one's flexibility also helps with balance and posture. Reduced mobility and persistent neck and back pain are two consequences of poor posture. Improved alignment and less tension on the back hips and hamstrings—two muscles that surround the spine—can be achieved with flexibility exercises. Furthermore, improved flexibility helps with balance, which is more crucial as men age and the likelihood of falls and associated injuries like fractures rises. Increasing flexibility with dynamic stretching or yoga poses can assist stabilize the body and lower the chance of falling.

Moreover, even in older men, flexibility training can improve athletic performance. Flexibility improves agility, power, and speed by enabling more effective movement patterns. Whether you like to play sports or participate in leisure activities, being flexible helps you give it your all and get the most out of these activities.

Think about combining static and dynamic stretching when adding flexibility exercises to your training regimen. Dynamic stretching combines movement into the stretches, whereas static stretching entails holding a stretch for an extended length of time. Both forms of stretching are advantageous and can be performed on their own or as part of a pre-workout warm-up.

It's crucial to remember that developing flexibility requires persistence and patience. Although you won't see results right away, daily practice will help you progressively gain more mobility and range of motion. It's important to pay attention to your body and avoid pushing yourself over your comfort zone because doing so can result in harm.

To sum up, men over 50 must practice flexibility if they want to keep their health and wellbeing at their best. It can support general physical and mental well-being, reduce the risk of injury, boost sports performance, and improve posture and balance. Including flexibility exercises in your fitness routine can significantly improve your quality of life as you age, provided you follow the right advice and are consistent with it.

Cool down Stretching Exercise.

Stretch your neck by sitting or standing upright. Till you feel a slight strain, slowly cock your head to one side and bring your ear close to your shoulder. Hold for a duration of 15-30 seconds. Continue on the opposite side.

Shoulder Stretch: Take a straight stance or sit up. Transform your right arm over your chest. Till your shoulder stretches, slowly bring your right arm up to your chest with your left hand. Hold for a duration of 15-30 seconds. Proceed with the left arm in the same manner. Stand with your feet shoulder-width apart for the chest opener. Make a handshake behind your back. Raise your arms slightly and extend them straight to open your chest. Hold for a duration of 15-30 seconds. Seated Forward Bend: Take a seat on the floor and extend your legs in front of you.Reach forward to your toes and hinge at the hips.Maintain a straight back.Hold for a duration of 15-30 seconds.Calf Stretch: Place your hands shoulder-height on a wall while facing it.Bend your front knee and take one straight step back.Feel the back leg's calf stretch as you slant forward a little.Hold for a duration of 15-30 seconds.Continue with the opposite leg.

Chapter2: Essential Stretches for Upper Body Mobility

Neck and Shoulder Stretches for Improved Posture

1. Neck Tilt:

- Sit or stand with erect backs.

- Tilt your head slowly to one side, bringing your ear close to your shoulder.

- After 15 to 30 seconds of holding, switch sides.

2. Neck Rotation:

- Turn your head slightly to one side while glancing over your shoulder.

- Repeat on the opposite side after holding for 15 to 30 seconds.

3. Neck Flexion:

- The back of your neck should extend as you slowly bring your chin up to your chest.

- Tent for fifteen to thirty seconds.

4. Shoulder Rolls:

- Raise your shoulders to your ears and then roll them in a circular motion back and forth.

- For 15 to 30 seconds, repeat.

<u>5. Shoulder Blade Squeeze:</u>

- Assume a proper seated or standing position.

- Squeeze and keep your shoulder blades together for ten seconds, then let go.

<u>6. Levator Scapula Stretch:</u>

- Tilt your head slightly to one side, bringing your shoulder to your ear.
- Put a slight pressure with your palm on the other side of your head.
- Switch sides after holding for 15 to 30 seconds.

<u>7. Extension of Upper Trapezius:</u>

- Bend your head to the side and place your ear against your shoulder.

- Pull your head ever so little with your hand.
- Switch sides after holding for 15 to 30 seconds.

8. Shoulder-crossing-body:

- Extend your arm over your chest.
- Carefully draw your arm toward your chest with your opposing hand.
- Switch sides after holding for 15 to 30 seconds.

9. Doorway Stretch:

- Place your arms shoulder-height while standing in a doorway.
- With your hands on the door frame, bend forward until you feel your shoulders and chest stretching.
- Tent for fifteen to thirty seconds.

The pectoral stretch is performed by standing with your hand at shoulder height on a wall or doorway.

Feel a stretch across your chest as you rotate your body away.

- Switch sides after holding for 15 to 30 seconds.

Chest and Upper Back Stretches for Better Mobility

<u>1. Squat-Cow Pose:</u>

- Begin by getting on your hands and knees.
- Breathe in and arch your back (cat pose).
- Let out a breath, arch your back (like a cow)

<u>2. Child's Pose:</u>

Extend your arms forward while kneeling on the mat and sitting back on your heels.

3. Pick Up the Needle:

- Start from all fours.
- Lower your shoulder to the mat by sliding one arm under the other.

4. Doorway Chest Opener:

- Raise your arms, stand in a doorway, and put your hands on the doorframe. Lean forward gently and open your chest.

5. Upper Back Twist:

- Cross your legs while sitting.
- Rotate your torso such that one hand is on the other knee.

6. Wall Angels:

- Make a snow angel gesture with your arms while standing up against a wall.

7. Lat Stretch:

- On a stability ball or bench, bend at the knees and extend your arms forward.

8. Thoracic Extension:

- Assume a heel-posing position and slowly arch your upper back with your hands behind your head.

9. Pec Stretch:

- Press onto the door frame while standing in a doorway with your arms raised to shoulder height.

10. Eagle Arms:

- Bend both elbows and bring palms together after crossing one arm under the other.

Arm and Forearm Stretches for Enhanced Range of Motion

1. Stretch Your Triceps:

- Bend the elbow as you extend your right arm overhead.
- Apply light pressure on the right elbow with your left hand.
- After holding for 15 to 30 seconds, swap sides.

2. Wrist Flexor Stretch:

- Raise your right arm out to the side, palm down.

- Lightly press down on the fingers with your left hand.
- After holding for 15 to 30 seconds, swap sides.

3. Stretch Your Wrist Extensor:

- Stretch out your right arm, palm up.
- Lightly press down on the hand's back with your left hand.
- After holding for 15 to 30 seconds, swap sides.
-

4. Forearm Flexor Stretch:

- Reach forward with your right arm.
- Press your fingers against the palm with your left hand.
- After holding for 15 to 30 seconds, swap sides.

5. Stretch Your Forearms:

- With your palm facing down, extend your right arm forward.
- Apply pressure to the fingers with your left hand.
- After holding for 15 to 30 seconds, swap sides.

6. Bicep Stretch:

- Raise your right arm and turn it palm up.
- Bring your hand to your upper back while bending your elbow.
- After holding for 15 to 30 seconds, swap sides.

7. Perform a shoulder stretch

- by crossing your right arm across your chest.

- Carefully draw the arm toward your chest with your left hand.
- After holding for 15 to 30 seconds, swap sides.

8. Overhead Triceps Stretch:

- Raise your right arm above your head and extend it down the middle of your back, bending the elbow.
- Apply light pressure on the right elbow with your left hand.
- After holding for 15 to 30 seconds, swap sides.

9. Shoulder and Neck Extension:

- Tilt your head so that your right ear is closer to your shoulder.
- Gently press with your right hand on the left side of your head.

- After holding for 15 to 30 seconds, swap sides.

10. Pronator Stretch:

- Reach forward with your right arm, palm down.
- Rotate the palm of your left hand toward your body while applying pressure to your fingers.
- After holding for 15 to 30 seconds, swap sides.

Chapter 3: Key Stretches for Lower Body Flexibility

Hip and Glute Stretches for Improved Hip Mobility

1. Stretch Your Hip Flexors:

- Make a 90-degree angle with your left foot in front as you kneel on your right knee.
- Feel the stretch in your right hip as you gently press your hips forward.
- After 30 seconds of holding, switch sides.

2. Pigeon Pose:

- Begin in plank posture, then draw your right leg towards your right palm.
- With your hips squared, extend your left leg behind you.

- As you lower your upper body toward the floor, your right glute should feel stretched.
- After 30 seconds of holding, switch sides.

3. Figure-Four Stretch while Sitting:

- Extend your legs while sitting on the floor.
- Maintaining a straight back, cross your right ankle over your left knee.
- Feel for a stretch in your right hip as you gently apply pressure to your right knee.
- After 30 seconds of holding, switch sides.

4. Butterfly Stretch

- Assume a seated position with your knees bent outward and your soles together.
- While keeping your feet planted, nudge your knees toward the ground.
- Sensate the stretch in your hips and inner thighs.

5.Hip Circles:

- Place your feet shoulder-width apart.
- Move your hips in a clockwise and counterclockwise circular motion.
- Work in each direction for 30 seconds.

6. Lizard Pose:

- Step your right foot outside of your right hand while starting from a plank position.
- Drop your hips till your right hip feels really stretched.
- After 30 seconds of holding, switch sides.

7. Standing Forward Bend:

- Place your feet hip-width apart, bend at the hips, and extend your arm to touch the ground.

- Feel the stretch in your glutes and hamstrings while maintaining a slight bend in your knees.

8. Seated Hip Stretch:

- Sit with your legs straight out in front of you.
- Hug your left knee toward your chest while crossing your right ankle over it.
- Your right hip should feel stretched.
- After 30 seconds of holding, switch sides.

9. Clamshell Stretch:

- Bend your knees while lying on your side.
- While keeping your feet together, stretch your outer hip and open your top knee.
- After holding for 15 seconds, swap sides.

10. Wall Hip Flexor Stretch

- Place your right foot on the wall behind you while standing facing a wall.
- Feel the stretch in your right hip as you lean forward while maintaining a straight back leg.
- After 30 seconds of holding, switch sides.

Hamstring and Quadriceps Stretches for Better Leg Flexibility

1. Hamstring Extension While Standing:

- Pace yourself hip-width apart.
- Maintain a straight back as you hinge at your hips and extend down towards your toes.
- Hold for 15 to 30 seconds, allowing your hamstrings to stretch.

2. Seated Hamstring Stretch:

- Extend your legs while sitting on the floor.
- Maintain a flat back while reaching forward toward your toes.
- Tent the stretch for a duration of 15-30 seconds.

3. Quad Stretch Forward Fold:

- Bend forward and reach for your toes while standing.
- To stretch your quads, bend one leg and bring your heel towards your glutes.
- Hold each leg for 15 to 30 seconds.

4. Lying Hamstring Stretch

- Start on your back, raise one leg, and grasp behind the calf or thigh.
- Maintain the other leg on the ground, either straight or bowed.
- Switch legs after 15 to 30 seconds of holding.

5. Lunge the Runner:

- Place one foot forward and begin in the lunge stance.

- Drop your hips and feel your quads and hip flexors stretch.

- Hold each leg for 15 to 30 seconds.

6. Chair Pose:

- Place your feet together, bend your knees, and drop your hips to resemble a chair.

- Maintain a stretched upper limb.

- Maintain for 15 to 30 seconds.

7. Pigeon Pose:

- Bring one knee to the same-side wrist while starting in a plank position.

- Straighten the opposite leg and extend it behind you.

- After 15 to 30 seconds of holding, switch sides.

8. Wall Hamstring Stretch

- Position your hips toward a wall while lying on your back.
- With the other leg bent or straight on the ground, extend one leg up against the wall.
- Switch legs after 15 to 30 seconds of holding.

9. Quad Stretch with Rotation:

- Bring your heel towards your glutes while standing on one leg and bending the other knee.
- Grab the foot by reaching back with the opposing hand.
- Hold each leg for 15 to 30 seconds.

10. Dynamic Leg Swings:

- To maintain balance, stand close to a wall or post.
- Swing a leg side to side, then back and forth.
- Repeat on each leg for ten to fifteen strokes.

Calf and Achilles Stretches for Injury Prevention and Flexibility

1. Calf Stretch Against a Wall:

- Place your hands on a wall while standing facing it.
- Take a step back and firmly plant your heel on the ground.
- Feel the stretch in your calf while maintaining a straight back leg.

2. Lounge Your Calf:

- Extend your legs while sitting.
- Gently bring a towel towards you by wrapping it around the ball of one foot.
- Sensate the strain in the leg's extended calf.

3. Dog Facing Downward:

- Take a plank stance to begin.
- While maintaining your heels on the ground, raise your hips toward the ceiling.
- Sensate the strain in your Achilles tendon and calves.

4. Calf Raises:

- Assume a level stance.
- Lift your heels up and then place them back down.
- Repeat to build stronger calves.

5. Achilles Stretch on a Stair

- Place your heels dangling over the edge of the stairwell as you stand there.
- Gently bring your heels down below the stair level.
- Sensate the Achilles tendon.

6. Toe Pulls:

- Sit with your toes pointed up and your legs extended.
- Point, flex, and tap your toes on the ground.
- Stretches and engages the calves.

7. Achilles towel stretch:

- Extend your legs while sitting.
- Gently bring a towel towards you by wrapping it around the ball of one foot.
- Sensate the Achilles tendon.

8. Resistance band calf stretches:

- Place a resistance band around one foot's ball and sit with your legs extended.
- Feel the strain in your calf as you gently pull the band towards you.

9. Nonsensical Heel Drops:

- Elevate your feet and dangle your heels.
- Lower heels gradually below the surface and then lift them back up.
- Enhances and extends the Achilles tendon.

10. Seated Toe Stretch:

- Extend your legs while sitting.
- While keeping your legs straight, reach for your toes.
- Sensate the strain in your Achilles and calves.

Chapter 4: Stretching for Balance and Core Strength

Stretching Exercises to Improve Balance and Stability

In order to improve general movement, avoid falls, and maintain proper posture, one must have adequate balance and stability. Exercising your limbs is a good approach to increase stability and balance. Enhancing flexibility, releasing tight muscles, and enhancing joint range of motion are all benefits of stretching that can lead to improved balance. We'll look at a few stretches in this post that are meant to improve stability and balance.

1. Hip Flexor Stretch: To begin, stand with one foot in front of you and the other behind you. Maintain a straight back and contract your core. Lean forward slowly, bending your front knee but maintaining a straight back leg. Your front thighs and hips ought should feel stretched. After 20 to 30 seconds, hold this posture, then swap sides.

2. Calf Stretch: Assume a standing position facing a wall or other stable vertical surface. With one foot planted firmly on the ground and your toes pointed forward, take a step back. Lean forward slowly, pressing against the wall but maintaining a straight back leg. Your calf muscle ought to feel stretched. For 20 to 30 seconds, hold this stretch on each leg.

3. Quadriceps Stretch: Bend your knee and raise one foot to your glutes while standing straight. Grasp your ankle with your other hand on the same side and pull it toward your body. The front of your thigh should stretch if you keep your knees close together. For 20 to 30 seconds, hold this stretch on each leg.

4. Stretch your hamstrings by perching on the edge of a bench or strong chair. With your toes pointing

upward and your heel lying on the floor, extend one leg forward. When you feel a stretch at the back of your thigh, slowly extend your hand forward while keeping your back straight. For 20 to 30 seconds, hold this stretch on each leg.

5. Glute Stretch: Lay flat on your back with your feet flat on the ground and both knees bent. Form a figure-four by crossing one ankle over the other knee. Feel for a stretch in the glute region by reaching behind the thigh of the lifted leg and pulling it slightly towards your chest. After 20 to 30 seconds of holding, switch sides.

6. Ankle Mobility Exercise: Place both feet flat on the floor while sitting tall in a chair. Elevate one foot off the ground and slowly spin your ankle clockwise for ten to fifteen seconds, followed by a counterclockwise rotation for an additional ten to fifteen seconds. Use the other foot to complete this exercise again.

7. Core Exercise: Weakness in the core is often associated with balance problems. Enhancing your general stability and balance can be achieved by strengthening your core muscles. To work the muscles in your core, try exercises like Russian twists, planks, side planks, and bird dogs.

It's important to remember to move slowly and deliberately during these stretching exercises—don't push yourself. To reap the greatest benefits from stretching, it's critical to breathe deeply and remain relaxed. Over time, including these exercises to your everyday regimen will help you become more stable and balanced.

It's crucial to perform balance-challenging workouts like Pilates, yoga, and tai chi in addition to these stretches. These exercises increase flexibility, strength, and body awareness in addition to improving balance.

Before beginning any new fitness regimen, always get advice from a medical expert or a trained fitness instructor, particularly if you have any prior injuries or medical concerns. Based on your unique demands, they can provide you tailored advice and adjustments.

You may increase your stability and balance, lower your chance of falling, and generally improve your quality of life by adding these stretching exercises to your daily workout regimen. Thus, give your body some time to stretch and strengthen it, then reap the rewards of better stability and balance.

Core Strengthening Stretches for a Stronger Midsection

1. Cobra Pose:

- Extend your legs while lying face down on the floor.
- Put your hands under your shoulder blades.
- To raise your upper body off the ground, straighten your arms and press your hands into the floor.
- Maintain your legs and hips down.
- Hold for ten to thirty seconds, then let go.

2. Child's Pose:

- Begin by bending over on your palms.
- Remain on your heels while keeping your big toes in contact.
- Reach your arms forward until your forehead meets the floor, lowering your torso between your thighs.
- Hold while inhaling deeply for 30 to 60 seconds.

3. Cat-Camel Stretch:

- Start from the hands and knees position.

- Take a breath, arching your back and lowering your head and tailbone as you do so.
- Release the air by burying your chin toward your chest and rounding your back downward.
- Do this flowing motion eight to ten times.

4. Lunge Twist:

- Place your feet hip-width apart.
- With your left hand on the ground, step your left foot back into a deep lunge.
- Twist your torso to the right and extend your right arm straight up toward the ceiling.
- Before repeating on the opposite side, hold for 20 to 30 seconds.

5. Supine Spinal Twist:

- Extend your legs while lying on your back.
- Bend and then cross your right knee over your left side.

- With your left arm out to the side, place your right hand on the ground.
- Take a few gentle steps to lower your right knee, then hold the position for a few seconds.
- Continue on the opposite side.

6. Side Plank Stretch:

- Begin by extending your legs while supporting your body on your right arm in the side plank position.
- Extend your left arm overhead, pointing it upwards.
- Hold each side for 20 to 30 seconds.

7. Standing Side Bend:

- Place your feet hip-width apart and stand tall.
- Spread your arms wide and firmly grasp your hands together.
- Feel the stretch down your left side as you slant slightly to the right.

- Hold for 20 to 30 seconds before moving to the opposite side.

8. Seated Forward Fold:

- Lie on your back and extend your legs in front of you.
- Extend your back and bend forward at the hips.
- Reach out while maintaining a straight back towards your shins or toes.
- Hold while inhaling deeply for 30 to 60 seconds.

9. Bridge Pose:

- Lie flat on your back with your feet flat on the floor and your knees bent.
- Lift your hips off the ground by pressing onto your heels.
- Press your arms down for support, overlapping your hands beneath your back.
- After 20 to 30 seconds of holding, carefully lower your body again.

10. Boat Pose:

- Bend your knees while sitting on the ground.
- Slightly slant backward and raise your feet off the ground while maintaining a tailbone balance.
- Straighten your arms in front of you and hold them parallel to the ground.
- Hold while using your core for 20 to 30 seconds.

During these stretches, keep an ear out for any pain or discomfort and pay attention to your body. The length and intensity should be gradually increased as you get more accustomed to the exercises.

Incorporating Yoga and Pilates into Your Stretching Routine

Every fitness or exercise regimen must include stretching. It aids in injury prevention, range of motion expansion, and flexibility improvement. While there are many other stretching methods, yoga and Pilates are particularly well-known for their capacity to increase balance and strength in the body as well as muscular stretching. This post will discuss how to include yoga and pilates in your stretching exercises and take advantage of all the health benefits they provide.

With an emphasis on the mind-body connection, yoga has been performed for thousands of years. It promotes both physical and mental wellness by combining a series of positions, breathing techniques, and meditation. Yoga offers a thorough method for stretching that addresses all of the main muscle groups. Yoga positions' gentle yet demanding nature helps you develop strength and stability while simultaneously stretching and lengthening your muscles.

You can begin incorporating yoga into your stretching regimen by performing a few yoga poses before or after your usual stretching session. Child's pose, downward dog, forward fold, and seated forward bend are a few of the well-liked yoga poses for flexibility. These positions work the hamstrings, hips, back, and shoulders, among other muscle groups. Maintain a calm and stable mind-set, concentrate on your breathing, and hold each pose for thirty to one minute. You can experiment with more difficult yoga poses as you go, which will test your strength and flexibility.

Conversely, Joseph Pilates created the low-impact Pilates exercise regimen. It emphasizes body awareness, body alignment, and core strength. Pilates exercises are done on a mat or with tools such as the Cadillac or reformer. Pilates' methodical and controlled movements enhance flexibility and coordination while strengthening and stretching the muscles.

You can include some Pilates movements that focus on particular muscle groups into your stretching regimen to incorporate Pilates. For instance, the Pilates roll-up exercise works wonders for strengthening the abdominal muscles and extending the spine. Stretching the hamstrings and strengthening the core are two excellent benefits of the Pilates leg pull front exercise. The Pilates swan exercise strengthens the posterior chain and stretches the muscles in the back, shoulders, and chest.

Seeking advice from a certified instructor who can teach you the proper form and technique is a good option if you're new to yoga or Pilates. They can assist you in determining the right degree and level of intensity for your stretching exercises. Additionally, you can stay consistent and advance in your practice by going to yoga or Pilates classes, which can offer a positive and encouraging environment.

There are many advantages to adding yoga and Pilates to your stretching exercises. Enhanced range of motion and flexibility are a few of the main benefits. improved endurance and strength of the muscles Enhanced bodily awareness and posture boosted general well-being and decreased tension and anxiety. Additionally, these techniques' cultivation of the mind-body link can aid in the development of mindfulness and calm.

Recall that maintaining consistency is essential to gaining the advantages of Pilates and yoga. For observable gains in your flexibility, strength, and general performance, try to practice three or four times a week. As with any workout regimen, pay attention to your body and adjust or advance the positions as necessary. You'll witness the transformational effects of adding Pilates and yoga to your stretching regimen with patience and commitment.

Chapter 5: Stretching Routines for Common Age-Related Conditions.

Addressing Joint Stiffness and Arthritis Through Stretching

Men over 50 frequently worry about arthritis and stiff joints. Joint wear and strain brought on by aging may cause stiffness, pain, and restricted movement. Stretching on a regular basis is one technique to help reduce these problems and enhance joint health.

Stretching is a helpful exercise that can help reduce stiffness in the joints and increase general flexibility. You can benefit from expanded range of motion, decreased pain and inflammation, improved blood circulation, and better joint function by adding stretching to your daily routine.

When doing stretches to treat joint stiffness and arthritis, it's critical to concentrate on certain body parts that are frequently impacted by these disorders. In general, your stretching program should focus mostly on the major joints, such as the spine, shoulders, hips, and knees. To find the best stretching exercises for your particular ailment, it's crucial to speak with a medical professional or a physical therapist.

Stretching Strategies for Managing Back Pain

All ages are commonly affected by back discomfort, but older men may find it especially difficult to manage. Our bones, muscles, and ligaments naturally deteriorate with age, making us more vulnerable to injury. Nonetheless, there are practical methods for handling back pain, and stretching exercises are essential for reducing soreness and increasing range of motion.

It's crucial to speak with a healthcare provider, such as a physical therapist or doctor, before beginning any stretching regimen. They can evaluate your unique situation and help you create a customized workout program. They are able to pinpoint any underlying problems and suggest activities that are tailored to your individual pain locations.

These are some stretching techniques that are especially helpful in treating back pain in older men; however, because we have already discussed this exercise, allow me to repeat it for maximum benefit.

1. <u>Start with gentle full-body stretches:</u> Start with stretches that target your entire body. These can include side bends, arm circles, and shoulder rolls as well as neck stretches. Try to progressively extend the range of motion without generating any discomfort.

2. Lower back stretches: Pay particular attention to stretching the quadratus lumborum and erector spinae, two muscles in the lower back. The knee-to-chest stretch is a quick and efficient stretch. With one leg bent and the other foot still on the floor, carefully raise one knee to your chest while lying on your back. After holding the stretch for 20 to 30 seconds, switch to the other side.

3. Hamstring stretches: Back pain may be exacerbated by hamstring tightness. Place one leg straight out in front of you while sitting on the edge of a chair or other stable surface to stretch them. Lean forward from the hips while maintaining a straight back until you feel a slight stretch in the back of your leg. After 20 to 30 seconds of holding, switch legs.

4. Hip stretches: It's crucial to stretch your hip flexors on a regular basis since they support your lower back in a big way. The standing quad stretch is one useful exercise. Use a chair or a wall as support when standing. Bend one knee and grip your ankle with your rear hand. When you feel a stretch in the front of your thigh, pull your ankle toward your glutes. After 20 to 30 seconds of holding, switch legs.

5. Exercises to strengthen your core: A strong core can support your spine and lower your chance of developing back discomfort. Include exercises like planks, bridges, and pelvic tilts that work the muscles in your abdomen. These workouts support proper posture and spine stability while doing daily tasks.

Don't forget to move slowly and deliberately through each stretch, without bouncing or abrupt movements. Try to stretch every day, or at least a few times a week, to keep your muscles loose and flexible.

Apart from stretching, several lifestyle modifications can aid in the management of back discomfort. A stronger and more resilient back can be achieved by maintaining a healthy weight, exercising regularly, and adopting excellent posture. Examples of aerobic exercises include walking and swimming. It's also critical to pay attention to your body and abstain from actions that make your pain worse.

Seeking medical assistance is vital if your back discomfort worsens or persists despite stretching and lifestyle improvements. A medical practitioner can assess your problem, do diagnostic testing as needed, and suggest additional treatment options, such as prescription drugs for physical therapy or, in certain situations, surgery.

In summary, treating back pain in older men calls for a multifaceted strategy that incorporates strengthening the core, stretching exercises that target particular muscle groups, and leading a healthy lifestyle. You can improve your quality of life, lessen discomfort, and increase flexibility by adopting these techniques into your everyday practice. Never forget to get medical advice before beginning any workout program to make sure it's safe and appropriate for your situation.

Stretching for Improved Circulation and Reduced Muscle Soreness

Stretching is a healthy habit that helps improve blood flow and lessen aching in the muscles. Stretching has several health benefits for the body when done correctly and consistently, making you feel more energized and at ease.

A major advantage of stretching is that it promotes better blood circulation. Your body's muscles and tissues become longer and more relaxed when you stretch them. By doing this, the blood can circulate through the body more effectively, providing the muscles with vital nutrients and oxygen. Improved circulation can also help the muscles rid themselves of waste products from metabolism, which lessens the chance of tired and aching muscles.

Moreover, stretching can relieve tension and pain in the muscles. Muscle tension can occur after physical exertion or periods of inactivity. Stretching can release any stored tension and assist in returning the muscles to their normal length. You can improve your flexibility and lower your chance of injury or muscle imbalances by stretching on a regular basis.

Stretching exercises are another way to increase joint range of motion. For joints to work correctly, a combination of muscles, ligaments, and tendons are needed. Joint mobility may be restricted and the risk of injury may rise when these structures are rigid or inflexible. You can increase your range of motion and lessen the strain on the joints themselves by stretching and lengthening the muscles surrounding them.

Stretching can also help to improve body alignment and posture. Overly taut or unbalanced muscles might result in postural abnormalities like forward-leaning heads or rounded shoulders. Frequent stretching can help to correct these muscular imbalances, promoting better alignment and posture. Maintaining good posture can ease discomfort and improve general health by reducing stress on the spine and other joints.

Stretching has advantages for the body, but it can also improve mental health. Stretching and paying attention to your body will help you feel more relaxed and less stressed. Stretching can be a mindful exercise that helps you become more aware of your body and the current moment. Those with hectic or stressful lives may find this to be especially helpful.

It's crucial to carry out the stretches correctly if you want to make sure you get the most out of them. Here are some pointers to remember:

1. Warm up before stretching: You can get your body temperature up and your muscles ready for stretching by jogging or walking, which are low-impact cardiovascular exercises.

2. Stretch all main muscle groups: Take care to stretch your arms, shoulders, back, legs, and hips, among other key muscle groups in your body.

3. Maintain stretches for the proper amount of time: Try to maintain each pose for 15 to 30 seconds. Steer clear of bouncing or jerking motions since these can cause harm.

4. Breathe deeply: To help your body relax and maximize the benefits of your stretches, inhale deeply while you perform them.

<u>5. extend both sides of your body equally:</u> Make sure you extend both sides of your body equally to preserve symmetry and balance.

<u>6. Stretch frequently:</u> When it comes to stretching, consistency is essential. To get the most out of stretching exercises, try to work them into your regular schedule.

It is crucial to remember that stretching shouldn't ever hurt or be uncomfortable. Stretching should be done gently if you feel any pain, or you should see a medical practitioner.

Chapter 6: Advanced Stretching Techniques for Optimal Performance

Dynamic Stretching for Warm-Up and Athletic Performance

<u>1. Leg Swings:</u>

- To maintain balance, stand close to a wall or other solid support.
- Make a controlled, fluid action with one leg swinging forward and backward.
- Increase the range of motion progressively with each swing.
- Make ten to fifteen swings with each leg.

2. Arm Circles:

- Extend your arms straight out to the sides while standing with your feet shoulder-width apart.
- Using your arms, make little circles that progressively get bigger.
- The circles then rotate in the opposite way after a few turns.
- Proceed in each direction for ten to fifteen circles.

3. Walking Lunges:

- Place your feet hip-width apart and stand tall to begin.
- Lean your torso forward to create a lunge position, extending your right leg.
- In order to execute the next lunge, step off with your right foot and extend your left leg.
- As you switch legs, remember to maintain a straight back and a front knee that is in line with your ankle.
- Lunge ten to twelve times on each leg.

4. High Knees:

- Place your feet hip-width apart while standing.
- To start, jog stationary while raising your knees as high as you can, one at a time.
- Maintain your upper body upright and your core active.
- Keep going for 30 to 60 seconds.

<u>5. Butt Kicks:</u>

- Place your feet hip-width apart while standing.
- Jog stationary, striving to touch your glutes with your heels as you kick them up behind you.
- Maintain your upper body upright and your core active.
- Keep going for 30 to 60 seconds.

Do not forget to begin these stretches slowly and build the intensity over time. Never ignore your body's signals to quit if you experience any pain or discomfort.

Proprioceptive Neuromuscular Facilitation (PNF) Techniques

In sports training and rehabilitation, proprioceptive neuromuscular facilitation (PNF) techniques are a popular class of stretching and strengthening exercises. In order to increase muscle coordination, strength, and range of motion, PNF approaches entail activating specific muscles and motions.

Dr. Herman Kabat and Margaret Knott, a physiotherapist, established the PNF concept in the 1940s. They discovered that specific muscle activation and movement patterns can enhance the neuromuscular system's reaction, improving functional skills.

Three fundamental concepts underpin PNF techniques: rhythmic initiation, autogenic inhibition, and reciprocal inhibition.

A muscle group that is activated during reciprocal inhibition is relaxed in the opposite muscle group. For instance, the triceps would contract but the biceps would remain relaxed while the elbow is bent. This idea supports stable joints and balanced muscular activity.

A muscle group contracts and then relaxes as a result of autogenic inhibition. This method aims to lengthen and enhance the range of motion of the muscles. The Golgi tendon organs, which are situated at the muscle-tendon junction, are stimulated by the contraction, and this causes the central nervous system to send signals that permit relaxation and greater flexibility.

A technique called rhythmic initiation is employed to progressively start a movement. It entails moving from a passive range of motion to an active range of motion with assistance, and then engaging in the movement actively. The recruitment and coordination of the muscles used in the movement are improved by this development.

PNF approaches are frequently applied in a variety of clinical contexts, such as sports training facilities and physical therapy offices. They can be used on patients with a variety of ailments, including post-surgical rehabilitation, neurologic impairments, and musculoskeletal disorders.

The following are a few PNF approaches that are frequently employed:

1. Contract-Relax (CR) approach: Under this approach, a specific muscle group isometrically contracts, and then the same muscle group is passively stretched. This method aims to increase the muscle's capacity for relaxation and flexibility.

2. Hold-Relax (HR) Technique: The HR technique is an isometric contraction of a target muscle group, much as the CR technique. At the conclusion of the range of motion, though, a static hold is used rather than a passive stretch. The goal of this technique is to increase the muscle's capacity to withstand an extended posture.

3. Combination of Isotonics (CIT): This method strengthens and enhances control over a particular range of motion by combining concentric and eccentric muscle contractions. One way to enhance upper limb strength and coordination is to alternate between bicep curls, which is a concentrated contraction, and tricep extensions, which is an eccentric contraction.

4. Slow Reversal (SR) Technique: To increase control and stability, this technique alternates between isometric contractions in opposing muscle groups. Enhancing knee joint stability can be achieved, for instance, by tightening the hamstrings and quadriceps against resistance.

5. Agonist Contract (AC) or Rhythmic Stabilization (RS) Technique: In these methods, one muscle group is isometrically contracted while resistance is provided by the opposite muscle group. These methods are frequently applied to enhance neuromuscular control and joint stability.

It is imperative to remember that PNF procedures must be used under the direction and supervision of a licensed healthcare provider, such as a certified trainer or physical therapist. They are able to modify the methods to suit specific requirements and guarantee correct application to avoid harm.

PNF methods are an effective tool for sports training and recuperation, to sum up. By employing particular movement patterns and muscle activation, they seek to enhance muscular coordination, strength, and range of motion. PNF procedures, when applied correctly and guided, can aid in injury recovery, improve sports performance, and boost general functioning abilities.

Incorporating Stretching into a Comprehensive Exercise Program

An all-encompassing fitness regimen must include stretching. Enhancing flexibility lowers the chance of injury, increases athletic performance, and advances general wellbeing. Stretching exercises can have a big impact on your fitness journey when added to your workout regimen.

Numerous stretching methods, such as proprioceptive neuromuscular facilitation (PNF) stretching, dynamic stretching, ballistic stretching, and static stretching, are frequently employed. Every approach has advantages of its own and ought to be used in particular circumstances.

The most popular type of stretching is called static stretching, and it is holding a stretch for an extended amount of time—usually 15 to 60 seconds. This kind of stretching works well for lengthening muscles and improving general flexibility. In order to assist relax the muscles and avoid pain after a workout, it is frequently employed as a cool-down exercise. Toe touches, hamstring stretches, and shoulder stretches are a few types of static stretches.

On the other hand, dynamic stretching entails carefully extending and contracting various body components across their whole range of motion. Stretching like this is especially helpful for pre-exercise or pre-competitive events. Dynamic stretching promotes joint mobility, boosts performance, and helps the muscles receive more blood flow. Walking lunges, leg swings, and arm circles are a few types of dynamic stretches.

A more complex type of stretching called ballistic stretching includes jerking or bouncing motions.

Stretching like this should be done carefully because improper execution increases the chance of damage. Athletes and anyone who need a high degree of flexibility for their activities, like dancers or gymnasts, are the main users of ballistic stretching.

Isometric contractions and passive stretching are combined in PNF stretching. It is frequently carried out with a partner's or physical therapist's assistance. PNF stretching targets particular muscle groups and improves neuromuscular coordination, which can assist increase flexibility. After an injury, this method is frequently applied in rehabilitation settings to restore range of motion.

The following recommendations should be taken into account when adding stretching to your workout regimen:

1. <u>Warm up your muscles before stretching</u>: It's important to warm up your muscles before beginning any stretching activities. Light cardiovascular exercises, such jogging or cycling for five to ten minutes, can help achieve this. Warming up helps the muscles receive more blood and gets them ready for stretching.

2. <u>Stretch all main muscle groups</u>: Make sure to include stretches that concentrate on all of your body's major muscle groups. Your arms, shoulders, back, hips, and legs are all included in this. Reduced flexibility and muscular imbalances might result from ignoring specific muscle groups.

3. <u>Hold the stretch</u>: Give each stretch a 15–60-second hold when doing static stretching exercises. Steer clear of bouncing or jerking motions since these can result in strained muscles. Rather, concentrate on a slow, continuous stretch.

4. Breathe deeply and relax: As you stretch, keep in mind to relax your muscles and take deep breaths. Keep in mind that tensing up or holding your breath can reduce the stretch's effectiveness.

5. extend both sides evenly: It's critical to extend your body equally on both sides. Make sure to repeat any stretches you perform on one side on the other. This promotes symmetry and equilibrium in the growth of your muscles.

6. Stretch frequently: It's critical to stretch frequently to observe discernible increases in flexibility. Consider adding stretching exercises to your regular routine and try to get in at least three or four days a week.

7. Pay attention to how your body feels: When you stretch, pay attention to how it feels. Ease off the stretch or adjust it to a comfortable level if you feel pain or discomfort. Never push yourself above your comfort zone when stretching since it could hurt.

It's crucial to combine stretching exercises with other elements of a thorough fitness program in addition to adding them to your training regimen. Exercises for the heart, muscles, and balance and coordination are included in this. These several components can be combined to create a comprehensive and successful exercise regimen.

In summary, stretching is an essential part of a thorough fitness regimen. It increases range of motion, boosts athletic performance, lowers injury risk, and advances general wellbeing. You may maximize the advantages of stretching and make the most of your fitness journey by including stretching exercises in your training regimen and adhering to the previously mentioned suggestions. Thus, prioritize stretching to get more flexibility and enhance your physical performance.

Conclusion.

In conclusion, a healthy lifestyle must include the full range of motion stretches recommended for men over 50. Men can enhance their flexibility, mobility, posture, and general well-being by stretching on a regular basis. Men over 50 should prioritise stretching activities that target age-related problems like reduced range of motion, muscle tightness, and stiff joints.

Men over 50 should incorporate a variety of stretches into their stretching exercises to target various muscle groups and body parts. This could involve mobility drills, dynamic stretches, and static stretches. It is crucial to begin with a mild warm-up in order to enhance blood circulation and prime the muscles for stretching.

Men over 50 might get several benefits from adding regular stretching into their routine. Stretching can help release tension and soreness in the muscles, lower the chance of injury, and enhance stability and balance. Additionally, it can improve general physical performance, which will facilitate and improve daily tasks.

Furthermore, stretching activities are beneficial for mental health. They can ease stress, encourage relaxation, and enhance concentration. Men over 50 may also use it as an opportunity to give self-care a high priority and set aside time for their own physical and emotional well-being.

It's critical to pay attention to your body's signals and refrain from straining past a comfortable range of motion during stretching. To guarantee correct form and safety when executing stretches, speaking with a licensed fitness instructor or medical practitioner is advised.

In conclusion, the full range of motion stretches recommended for men over 50 are a vital resource for preserving and enhancing physical health and general wellbeing. Men can support their ageing gracefully and maintain flexibility, mobility, and vitality by including stretching into their daily routine. Thus, make the decision to stretch regularly and enjoy all the advantages it provides for leading a happy and healthy lifestyle.